ESSENTIAL OILS FOR ARTHRITIS

CHOOSING A NATURAL APPROACH TO ELIMINATE
ARTHRITIS

By Tonny M Ford, RN, BSN, PHN.

© **2015**

Essential Oils

FOR ARTHRITIS

CHOOSING A NATURAL APPROACH TO ELIMINATE ARTHRITIS

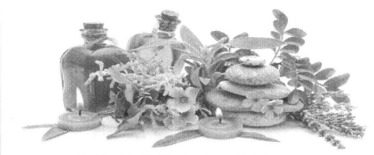

TONNY M FORD, RN, BSN, PHN

essentialoilRN.net

DISCLAIMER

This book is not intended as a substitute for the medical advice of physicians. The reader should regularly consult a physician in matters relating to his/her health and particularly with respect to any symptoms that may require diagnosis or medical attention.

The information provided in this book is designed to provide helpful information on the subjects discussed. This book is not meant to be used, nor should it be used, to diagnose or treat any medical condition. For diagnosis or treatment of any medical problem, consult your own physician. The publisher and author are not responsible for any specific health or medical needs that may require medical supervision and are not liable for any damages or negative consequences from any treatment, action, application or preparation, to any person reading or following the information in this book. References are provided for informational purposes only and do not constitute endorsement of any websites or other sources. Readers should be aware that the websites listed in this book may change.

within this book are for clarifying purposes only and are the owned by the owners themselves, not affiliated with this document.

We highly recommend that you consult a doctor and other trained clinicians before using essentials oils or anything that can affect your health. Your doctor is the only one who knows the true story of your health and can give your better professional help.

BONUS GIFT!!

As a way of saying thank you for purchasing our book, we have included a free 140 page exclusive pdf report on **essential oils guide**. We believe that that the value in this report will enrich your life abundantly. As a subscriber, you will the first to get a new free eBooks before anyone else! If you have any questions, please contact us at support@essentialoilrn.net

Click here to download your free bonus eBook

http://www.essentialoilrn.net/thanks/

TABLE OF CONTENTS

Making Sense of it All

Conclusion

I want to thank you and congratulate you for getting the book, *"Essential Oils for Arthritis – Choosing a Natural Approach To Eliminate Arthritis"*.

This book contains proven steps and strategies on how to choose essential oils and apply them when seeking to treat arthritis.

This book looks at the potential of treating arthritis with natural approaches rather than traditional medicine and contains an exhaustive list of appropriate essential oils that contain qualities that will address the at best, uncomfortable and at worst, painful symptoms of arthritis. Essential oils are a popular method when adopting natural approaches. The use of essential oils in this way for arthritis has changed people's lives and provided solutions where conventional medicine has not.

By understanding the background and properties of all of these oils and supplementary ingredients, arthritis sufferers can now make more informed choices about how to deal with their condition and can understand its cause and the best treatments for them. The ability to combine different ingredients will empower the arthritis sufferer to make informed choices on those that are suitable for them, giving them the flexibility that traditional doctors and medicines have not prescribed.

By reading this guide, the user will become an expert on essential oils for arthritis and know how to get the best out of each one.

Thanks again for purchasing this book, I hope you enjoy it!

CHAPTER 1

ARTHRITIS

Arthritis is an illness that affects the joints in the human body, causing sufferers pain and stiffness. A common disease, arthritis affects millions of people all over the world. It can emerge among any age group, including children and young persons less than 18 years of age; but its presence in older people over the age of 50, is more prevalent.

There are over a hundred types of arthritis that can be developed but the two most common forms are osteoarthritis and rheumatoid arthritis.

OSTEOARTHRITIS

Osteoarthritis develops when the smooth cartilage (or connective tissue) that lines the joints of the bones starts to thin. Without this protective layer, the joints' bones start rubbing together, which can cause swelling and the formation of osteophytes. Osteophytes are the formation of 'bone spurs' or projections that form along the margins of the bone. The sensation felt is that of stiffness and it is usually painful. The most commonly affected areas are the knees, elbows, hips, spine and hands.

This is the most common form of arthritis as it occurs from the normal wear and tear of bones or namely joints, hence it being known as an older person ailment, for those over the age of 65. It is thought that at least one in every two persons would develop osteoarthritis in the knee eventually in their life. Other causes of osteoarthritis may be obesity i.e. undue pressure on the joints, a previous joint injury, overuse of the joints, weak thigh muscles and also genially, if the family has a history of arthritis.

Severity can vary depending on each case and can occur in different joints, each generating their own symptoms. Sufferers of arthritis usually complain of symptoms after resting periods, such as in the morning when they have woken after a night of sleep. Symptoms may be particularly bad if sufferers endure activity for extended periods of time, but they do not suddenly appear, but rather take time to develop.

Stiffness is often temporary, and normality is often restored if the patient becomes active again. Sufferers may hear clicking sounds when they bend whatever joint is affected, and there tends to be inflammation, which causes the pain that gradually gets worse throughout the day.

Knees, hips, feet and hands

If one suffers from arthritis of the hip, the pain tends to be felt in the groin or gluteus and the back of the knee and thigh. If one suffers form arthritis of the knee, then one would be able to feel the joints grinding against each other when that joint is moving. Arthritis in the fingers means that fingers will feel tender and pain is felt in the thumb. Likewise arthritis in the feet will manifest in tenderness and pain felt in the big toes while pain may also be felt in the ankles.

Managing Symptoms

This stiffness or pain affects sufferer's daily lives because ordinary tasks become difficult. Particularly when hands or other joints in the upper body are affected, opening tins, changing linen and using the computer become incredibly painful and difficult or not possible at all. If joints such as the feet, knees and hips are affected then mobility is severely impacted, slowing the person down substantially.

On one hand, as osteoarthritis develops with time and the normal wear and tear of the body, many believe there is no point in managing the effects of arthritis. However, some measures could be taken to manage the damage that can be caused to joints as well as the symptoms i.e. pain, mobility and flexibility, so that sufferers can enjoy a better quality of life or less impediment.

Indirect impacts

As well as the direct affects of osteoarthritis such as stiffness and pain, it can have some indirect health impacts, which are caused by its symptoms i.e. pain and lack of movement and even side effects from prescribed medicine. Less mobility means increased weight and possible obesity, leading to diabetes, increased blood pressure and heart conditions. There is also an increased risk of falling and fractures due to the weakening of the muscles or even from faintness caused by some medications.

Causes

While osteoarthritis is mostly caused by long-term wear and tear, it is now seen as a joint disease and can be caused by other factors. It has been genially linked for example, a person may have an inherited condition whereby their body is under-producing collagen - collagen is the protein that forms the cartilage; or an inherited condition whereby joints do not align properly so they grind together and wear down the cartilage early. A gene related to pain sensitivity is also greater in those who suffer from osteoarthritis of the knee than anyone else. Obesity or overweight persons have more propensity to developing osteoarthritis as well due to the added pressure that is being applied to the knees and hips and over time this causes the cartilage in the joints to deteriorate, quicker than in those of normal weight. Excess fat can also produce cytokines, which are chemicals that cause inflammation, which is another reason that joints suffer in these persons. Another development of osteoarthritis is caused through the overuse of joints either through repetitive movements over long periods of time such as heavy lifting or monotonous and automated jobs or repeated injuries such as might be suffered by athletes.

There are other slightly obscure causes of arthritis, which cause chemical or hormone imbalances, therefore, seeking advice is suggested when symptoms start displaying.

RHEUMATOID ARTHRITIS

Rheumatoid arthritis is another common form of this disease and is more likely to be experienced by women. It is caused by a compromised immune system, which targets tissue lining the joints in the body known as the synovial membrane. The membrane covering the joint becomes inflamed and swells, stretching the cavity that is holding the joints in place. After the swelling goes down, the cavity does not restore to its initial position and the joint is not held in place. This makes the joints rest abnormally causing what is known as rheumatoid arthritis. It means that joints feel painful and stiff.

Causes

An abnormal immune system was mentioned, however, the causes of this abnormal development of the immune system is not fully known but may be linked to geniality, hormone balance or environment. Genes for example, have been attributed, as there is scientific evidence to show the presence of certain genes e.g. HLA shared epitope, STAT4, C5 and TRAF1, are more likely to develop rheumatoid arthritis because these genes control the immune system. There may be other causes such as infectious bacteria and viruses; female hormones obesity and trauma have also been linked to this particular form of arthritis. Some environmental factors that have been linked are passive smoking, pollution, insecticides and exposure to certain minerals (in large or extended proportions).

Symmetrical impact and symptoms

Just like osteoarthritis, the condition tends to affect joints such as the knees, wrists, hands, ankles and feet on both sides of your body i.e. left and right side. The symptoms include stiffness and pain in the joints, aching muscles, low blood count and a propensity to fever. As with osteoarthritis, stiffness is felt greatest after periods of rest, particularly in the morning after the night's sleep and pain can be felt greatest towards the end of the day.

Whereas osteoarthritis will affect older people in the majority of cases, rheumatoid arthritis tends to hit persons (mostly women) between 30 and 50 years of age. How rheumatoid arthritis affects you depends on the severity and on which joints are affected. It is quite common in the feet and hands as small joints tend to be affected initially. Inflammation can cause joints, such as in the toes and fingers, to grow and therefore, freeze into one position, so the sufferer cannot use that joint properly. It can also cause deformities such as hammertoe - the curling upwards of the toe – or the angling of the big toe towards the second toe. This can also cause corns to develop on top of the toes. It can lead to flatfoot if the arthritis reaches the middle of the foot, which can lead to the balls of the feet slipping forward also – this is very painful and felt every time the arthritis sufferer walks. At times it can extend to the hind foot, making the heel bend outwardly, which makes walking again very difficult and the uneven steps taken mean more calluses, corns and other viral foot conditions are likely to develop plus the formation of fleshy nodules around the joints.

Early diagnosis of rheumatoid arthritis makes it easier to manage and may prevent some of those deformities from developing. Advice as soon as you develop symptoms is advised.

Other Types

Osteoarthritis and rheumatoid arthritis are the most common forms of arthritis but as mentioned there are over 100 types. Diagnosis as soon as you start exhibiting symptoms or stiffness and pain around your joints is advised, then proper diagnosis will determine the appropriate treatment. Some other types of arthritis are as follows: -

Enteropathic arthritis – this is associated with inflammatory bowel disease (IBD) and tends to affect the limbs and spine.

Gout – this is caused by excessive uric acid in the body. While it can occur in any of the joints, it tends to occur in the big toe.

Lupus – this is an autoimmune disease, meaning that the immune system is attacking itself. As well as attacking joints, it can actually affect many parts of the body.

Psoriatic arthritis – this is prevalent in persons with psoriasis and causes inflammation of the joints.

CHAPTER 2

NATURAL APPROACHES VS. MEDICINAL

Arthritis is a very old condition and traces back to the year 4500 BC. As such, the use of natural remedies was well in use and an effective way to treat this ailment, although not necessarily to cure it. Some of these natural remedies are recommended by the medical practitioners themselves and in some cases may provide greater relief.

In the first instance, however, it is important to get correct diagnosis from the doctor and an overview of natural treatment with a special focus on essential oils will be looked at.

Diagnosis

If you are exhibiting symptoms of stiffness and pain around your joints, visit your GP. They will want to know information on your family health history as well as your personal medical history.

It is important you accurately describe symptoms to your doctor, such as when you started to experience pain and stiffness in your joints, which areas in particular, how this has affected different activities in your day, any medical problems and any current medicinal prescription. They may conduct some tests under a physical examination such as seeing how well the joints move and look for any signs of joint damage, abnormalities in alignment including that of the neck and spine. They may also extract joint fluid to test for signs of deterioration or perform an X-ray or MRI.

Prescriptive and traditional treatments

In order to manage symptoms, your doctor may prescribe pain relief and anti-inflammatory medication. Commonly prescribed medicines include:

Analgesics – this is composed of tramadol, narcotics and acetaminophen.

Non-steroidal anti-inflammation drugs (NSAIDs) – this is composed of aspirin, celecoxib, ibuprofen and naproxen.

Corticosteroids – this is anti-inflammatory and comes in vaccine form, injected into the joint by a medical practitioner.

Hyaluronic acid – this is a natural fluid that is present in a normal functioning joint to act as a lubricant and shock absorber. This can be injected by a medical practitioner and replenishes that which has already broken down in joints.

Physical and occupational therapy – this means that specialist therapists will administer heat therapies and cold therapies and can assist with exercises or recommend the use of assisted devices e.g. scooters etc.

Joint replacement surgery – the replacement of affected joints with metal or plastic joint parts. This may be a last resort for arthritis sufferers with permanent damage that has had a significant impact on their lives.

Overall natural treatments

While prescriptive methods may work, even the doctor will recommend that you apply lifestyle adjustments to help you manage symptoms or prevent further damage.

These can include, weight reduction or maintaining an already healthy weight to alleviate pressure being placed on the joints. More exercise or physical activity can keep stiffness at bay. While your joints may hurt, in the long run it will help to ease the pain as long as exercise is not too strenuous. In particular, resistance and strength building exercises are recommended as this will help to build muscles around the joints, which actually eases the burden on them. Some cardio is also useful in order to maintain levels of physical activity and to maintain a healthy weight.

Stretching, yoga or tai chi is recommended for improved flexibility around the joints. It will not only lessen stiffness but also help reduce pain.

Something as simple as a positive attitude can also help to combat the symptoms of arthritis. This has to do with the immune system, as a bad immune system can cause rheumatoid arthritis. Positivity is said to boost the immune system and to help manage pain.

Natural and Alternative Therapies

The above example of natural methods ties in with holistic approaches to medicine.

Many people with arthritis adopt natural/ alternative therapies to address their symptoms to include nutritional supplements, hydrotherapy, acupressure/acupuncture and essential oils.

Holistic medicine takes into account both the mind and body of a person when approaching the healing process. It does not just look at a disease in isolation. As it is believed that the whole self is made up of interconnecting parts, where if one were affected, the impact would be felt on another.

The holistic approach takes into account all aspects of a person's life such as sleep pattern, diet, exercise, psychological problems, mental exertion or any other illnesses. This ties in with the advice given by many doctors and essential oils are part of this approach to therapy.

Essential Oils

Essential oils are oils extracted from plants and are so named as they hold the "essence" of the plant's fragrance. They are used in fragrances, soaps and other consumer products and are even used medicinally.

Although they have been used throughout history for medical purposes, their use went into decline until recently. Aromatherapy has now become popular, adopted by many looking at alternative and holistic medicine options and essential oils are an essential part of this. As such they are now used for a range of ailments including joint problems, usually diluted in something known as a 'carrier oil'; as oils themselves, they cannot be diluted in water. The aromatic compounds in the oil is said to have healing effects e.g. antiseptic or stress relief.

Essential oils can be derived from numerous source materials, a list of some of those known include:

Berries	Valerian	Juniper	Seeds	Almond
Anise	Buchu	Celery	Cumin	Nutmeg oil
Bark	Cassia	Cinnamon	Sassafras	Wood

Camphor	Cedar	Rosewood	Sandalwood	Agarwood
Rhizome	Galangal	Ginger	Leaves	Basil
Bay leaf	Buchu	Cinnamon	Common sage	Eucalyptus
Guava	Lemongrass	Melaleuca	Oregano	Patchouli
Peppermint	Pine	Rosemary	Spearmint	Tea tree
Thyme	Tsuga	Wintergreen	Resin	Benzoin
Copaiba	Frankincense	Myrrh	Flowers	Cannabis
Chamomile	Clary sage	Clove	Scented geranium	Hops
Hyssop	Jasmine	Lavender	Manuka	Marjoram
Orange	Rose	Ylang-ylang	Peel	Bergamot
Grapefruit	Lemon	Lime	Orange	Root

Essential Oils for Arthritis

Essential oils have been used by many to alleviate the symptoms of arthritis and some of its causes. Many essential oils have properties that can tackle inflammation, relieve pain and boost the immune system. The calming effects of some essential oils can also help sufferers maintain a balanced lifestyle, increasing positivity and energy to avoid stress or depression.

Holistic methods, including the use of essential oils, can really impact people's lives and have been shown to help arthritis sufferers, where traditional medicine has not had the effects hoped for.

It is important however, that arthritis sufferers always approach their GP for diagnosis and take their advice.

CHAPTER 3

THE BEST ESSENTIAL OILS FOR ARTHRITIS

BAY LEAF ESSENTIAL OIL

Bay leaf essential oil comes from the leaves of the bay tree, which is found in the Caribbean, although it has spread to other parts of the world.

The bay leaf was an important part of old Roman and Greek civilizations and was heavily used in their medicinal practices, while also being an important part of their culture, using it to form crowns for accomplished people such as Olympians, warriors and kings. It is also frequently used in cooking.

The chemical components contained in bay leaf essential oil includes: alpha-pinene, alpha-terpineol, beta-pinene, chavicol, eugenol, geranyl acetate, linalool, limonene, myrcene, methyl chavicol and neral.

Bay leaf essential oil for arthritis has many benefits including as an analgesic because it reduces pain, as a tonic as it boosts the immune system and as a sedative to generally reduce stress and relax sufferers of arthritic illnesses.

Caution should be applied for pregnant women and because of its content of euganol, it can cause skin irritation therefore, beware of overusing.

Blends well with:

Cedar wood essential oil, coriander essential oil, eucalyptus essential oil, geranium essential oil, ginger essential oil, juniper essential oil, lavender essential oil, lemon essential oil, orange essential oil, rose essential oil, rosemary essential oil, thyme essential oil and ylang ylang essential oil.

CEDAR WOOD ESSENTIAL OIL

Cedar wood essential oil comes from the wood of the cedar wood tree found throughout the world but predominantly cold climates.

As well as for the use as an essential oil, cedar wood has a lovely scent and is typically used for incense.

The chemical components of cedar wood essential oil include alpha-cedrene, beta-cedrene, cedrol, sesquiterpenes, thujopsene and widdrol.

The main health benefit of cedar wood essential oil is that it is an anti-inflammatory and is well-documented for its use on arthritis, it is a tonic that helps tighten muscles, which is very important for the relief of pressure on the joints and its use as a sedative helps to calm the mind and encourage a healthy and positive mindset.

It is advisable however, not to use cedar wood oil in large quantities as it can be an irritant to the skin. It is not advisable for pregnant women. It is also highly potent so cannot be ingested. If consumed it causes nausea, vomiting, thirst and damage to the digestive system.

Blends well with:

Bergamot essential oil, benzoin essential oil, cypress essential oil, cinnamon essential oil, frankincense essential oil, juniper essential oil, jasmine essential oil, lemon essential oil, lime essential oil, lavender essential oil, rose essential oil, neroli essential oil and rosemary essential oil.

CHAMOMILE ESSENTIAL OIL

Chamomile essential oil comes from the flowers of the chamomile plant found throughout the world. There are many types of chamomile plant but the Roman chamomile and German chamomile are the most common.

The use of chamomile has a long history and was first noted for its use in ancient Egypt for curing fever, cosmetic purposes and embalming pharaohs.

The chemical components in Roman chamomile essential oil include alpha-pinene, beta-pinene, camphene, caryophyllene, sabinene, myrcene, gamma-terpinene, pinocarvone, farsenol, cineole, propyl angelate and butyl angelate. (German chamomile is slightly different and contains azulene, alpha-bisabolol, bisabolol oxide-A & B and bisabolene oxide-A).

Chamomile essential oil for arthritis has many benefits including as an anti-inflammatory and sedative to reduce stress and to reduce inflammation that causes severe discomfort to arthritis sufferers. It is also anti-rheumatic and anti-phlogistic, which means it improves circulation and reduces toxins like uric acid found in some arthritis sufferers and reduces swelling. The added benefit of German chamomile is that it is a vasoconstrictor, which means it reduces blood pressure.

Chamomile is a very low risk essential oil and therefore, can be used by a wide range of arthritis sufferers. However, those with known allergies to chamomile should avoid it.

Blends well with:

Bergamot essential oil, clary sage essential oil, geranium essential oil, grapefruit essential oil, jasmine essential oil, lavender essential oil, lemon essential oil, lime essential oil, rose essential oil, tea tree essential oil and ylang-ylang essential oil.

CLARY SAGE ESSENTIAL OIL

Clary sage essential oil is made from clary sage herb's buds and leaves, which is abundant in Europe.

The name clary is derived from a Latin word meaning 'clear' as it was used by the Romans as eyewash. Further uses have been for in wine and beer to replace hops.

The chemical components of clary sage essential oil include clareol, alpha-terpineol, geraniol, linalyl acetate, linalool, caryophyllene, neryl acetate and germacrene-D.

Its use as an essential oil for arthritis is mostly as an anti-inflammatory. However, its calming and euphoric attributes also make it beneficial as part of a holistic approach to increasing a positive outlook as it is an anti-depressant, nervine, euphoric and sedative. It also works to reduce blood pressure, which can be a secondary symptom of arthritis.

Side effects and hazards of using clary sage are associated with its sedative nature and can enhance the intoxification affects of alcohol or drugs. A large amount of ingestion can result in headaches. Pregnant women and breastfeeding mothers should avoid use as not enough research has been done on the hormonal affects of this essential oil.

Blends well with:

> Frankincense essential oil, geranium essential oil, jasmine essential oil, juniper essential oil, lavender essential oil, lemon essential oil, lime essential oil, orange essential oil, pine essential oil and sandalwood essential oil.

CYPRESS ESSENTIAL OIL

Cypress essential oil comes from the stems, twigs and needles of the Cypress tree, found throughout the world.

The cypress tree has been generally popular for its wood as it has reputation for being strong and durable and therefore abundantly used in interior and exterior fittings.

The chemical components of cypress essential oil include alpha-pinene, beta-pinene, alpha-terpinene, bornyl acetate, cadinene, camphene, carene, cedrol, linalool, myrcene, sabinene, and terpinolene.

The health benefits of cypress essential oil for arthritis include as an anti-inflammatory as well as a hemostatic and styptic, which helps to improve blood circulation and remove toxins. Its benefits relating to the lowering of blood pressure and as a sedative are also useful.

The use of cypress essential oil is low risk but is advised against use for pregnant women.

Blends well with:

Lime essential oil, lemon essential oil, orange essential oil, bergamot essential oil, clary sage essential oil, frankincense essential oil, juniper essential oil, lavender essential oil, marjoram essential oil, pine essential oil, rosemary essential oil and sandalwood essential oil.

EUCALYPTUS ESSENTIAL OIL
Eucalyptus essential oil is made from the leaves on the eucalyptus tree found in Australia.

Its nativity to Australia meant it was used prolifically by aboriginal peoples and was treated as an all-encompassing cure. In fact due to its capacity to absorb a substantial amount of water, it was placed abundantly in marshy areas in order to clear up the soil and air.

The chemical components of eucalyptus essential oil include alpha-pinene, beta-pinene, alpha-phellandrene, 1,8-cineole, limonene, terpinen-4-ol, aromadendrene, epiglobulol, piperitone and globulol.

Eucalyptus essential oil is an anti-inflammatory and has substantial benefits for arthritis sufferers to relieve joint and muscle pain. It also is known for providing a refreshing and cooling effect, which can address mental exhaustion or stress, the relief of which is beneficial to helping curb symptoms of arthritis.

Eucalyptus essential oil can be toxic if it is taken in excessive quantities, therefore, it should be taken in moderation. Those with allergic sensitivities should also be cautious while using eucalyptus essential oil.

Blends well with:

> Cedar wood essential oil, frankincense essential oil, lavender essential oil, marjoram essential oil, rosemary essential oil and thyme essential oil.

FRANKINCENSE ESSENTIAL OIL

Frankincense essential oil is found in the gum or resin of Boswellia trees, mostly in the Arabian Peninsula and North Africa.

Frankincense got its fame from the Bible, in the story of the three wise men that took frankincense and myrrh to baby Jesus as their gifts. It is common and popular in the use of medicine.

The main chemical components of the frankincense essential oil include alpha-pinene, actanol, bornyl acetate, linalool, octyl acetate, incensole and incensyl acetate.

The main benefit of frankincense essential oil is as an anti-inflammatory and is common in the treatment of knee pain.

Frankincense essential oil should be avoided by pregnant women due to possible hormonal interference.

Blends well with:

> Lime essential oil, lemon essential oil, orange essential oil, benzoin essential oil, bergamot essential oil, lavender essential oil, myrrh essential oil, pine essential oil and sandalwood essential oil.

GINGER ESSENTIAL OIL

Ginger essential oil comes from the spice, ginger. It is found in southern China and now other parts of Asia and West Africa.

Ginger is a common spice used in cooking and has been associated typically with easing stomach problems.

The main chemical components of ginger include zingiberene, zingibain beta-sesquiphelandrene, ar-curcumene and gingerols.

The health benefits of ginger essential oil for arthritis, mostly come from zingibain as it is an anti-inflammatory and reduces pain and muscle aches.

While ginger is quite strong it is relatively safe, however, it is not recommended for use during pregnancy as there is some evidence of miscarriages if used in abundance. It is also not recommended for excessive use.

Blends well with:

Lemon essential oil, cedar wood essential oil, lime essential oil, eucalyptus essential oil, frankincense essential oil, geranium essential oil, rosemary essential oil, sandalwood essential oil, patchouli essential oil, myrtle   essential oil, bergamot essential oil, rosewood essential oil, neroli essential oil, orange essential oil and ylang-ylang essential oil.

GRAPEFRUIT ESSENTIAL OIL

Grapefruit essential oil comes from the citrus fruit, grapefruit and is found in places of sub-tropical climate such as Jamaica.

The grapefruit, when first discovered in the Caribbean, was named "the forbidden fruit" because it was a hybrid fruit that was thought to have been created when a Captain Shaddock brought pomello seeds to Jamaica.

The main chemical components of grapefruit essential oil include alpha-pinene, citronellal, decyl acetate, neryl acetate, myrcene, sabinene, linalool, limonene, geraniol and terpinenol.

The health benefits of grapefruit essential oil include it being a well-known stimulant and tonic that keeps circulation in order, which is of good use to those suffering from arthritis caused by deficiencies to their immune system. However, it has been noted that grapefruit essential oil is also beneficial in alleviating stiffness, which would provide some relief for arthritis.

In normal quantities, grapefruit essential oil would not have any particular side effects. However, large quantities may have effects on the hormones, therefore, it is best to avoid in excess. Pregnant women, breastfeeding mothers and those with breast cancer should avoid to air on the side of caution.

HELICHRYSUM ESSENTIAL OIL

Helichrysum essential oil is derived from a plant in the sunflower family. It can also be referred to as 'immortelle'.

The helichrysum flower and its use dates back to 4000 BC and has been noted for its use in traditional medicine; however it has also been noted for its use in cooking, particularly in Italy.

The main chemical compounds within helichrysum essential oil are 1,8-cineole, bicyclosesquiphellandrene, gamma-curcumene, alpha-amorphene and bicyclogermacrene.

Helichrysum essential oil is an anti-inflammatory and nervine. Therefore, its ability to reduce swelling in the joints can help arthritis sufferers. It can also be a relaxant and tackle stress.

Helichrysum essential oil can be toxic so it should not be ingested. The normal risks of being sensitive to helichrysum essential oil still applies and this oil should always be diluted with one of the carrier oils. There are no known effects to pregnant women or breastfeeding mothers but advice should be sought nonetheless before application.

Blends well with:

> Geranium essential oil, lavender essential oil, lime essential oil, orange essential oil, rose essential oil, sage essential oil and ylang-ylang essential oil.

JUNIPER ESSENTIAL OIL
Juniper essential oil is made from the needles and wood of the conferous plant, juniper.

One interesting fact regarding the history of juniper is that the Romans used to use it in Olympic events, as they believed it improved the stamina of athletes.

The chemical components within it include alpha-pinene, camphene, beta-pinene, sabinene, myrcene, alpha-phellandrene, alpha-terpinene, gamma-terpinene, cineole, beta-phellandrene, para-cymene, terpineol, bornyl acetate and caryophyllene, limonene, camphor, linalool, linalyl acetate, borneol and nerol.

Its benefits for arthritis sufferers include it being anti-rheumatic to help blood circulation and guard against toxins thus warding off harmful pathogens, including uric acid and thus useful for treating gout.

Advice suggests that the use of juniper essential oil should be avoided for pregnant women, breastfeeding mothers and persons with kidney stones as it can stimulate the uterine muscle. It is not particularly sensitive to the skin but some users may experience a reaction to it, therefore, it should be used in moderation. Its use is advised against for children also.

Blends well with:

Cedar wood essential oil, clary sage essential oil, cypress essential oil, geranium essential oil, grapefruit essential oil, lavender essential oil, lavandin essential oil, bergamot essential oil, lime essential oil and lemongrass essential oil.

LAVENDER ESSENTIAL OIL
Lavender essential oil is made from the flowers of the lavender plant, commonly grown. The

chemical components of lavender essential oil include linalool and linalyl acetate.

Lavender has historically been most commonly used as perfume, forming the base of perfumes and other scents with even the Egyptians using it to wrap their dead in.

Lavender has numerous benefits and is incredibly versatile, which makes it a popular choice as an essential oil in the treatment of psoriasis. Lavender essential oil is anti-inflammatory. It therefore aids arthritis sufferers in alleviating inflammation around their joints. Lavender essential oil possesses calming properties as well. Therefore, if diffused into the air, the aroma can relax the mind. This can help sufferers to sleep, which is one way of alleviating stress symptoms, which are never conducive to all round good health and wellness of body required to fight any disease. It can also target the nervous system, which again targets nerves and anxiety. Lavender essential oil also has anti-bacterial and ant-viral qualities, occasionally a cause of some arthritis. As mentioned, the immune system in arthritis sufferers is often affected, which means healthy cells are often mistaken for pathogens. Using lavender essential oil, therefore will help arthritis sufferers fight disease.

Caution should be applied in the use of lavender essential oil by children, those who are pregnant and mothers who are breastfeeding. Mostly, there is not enough evidence for the possible side effects on this group of individuals. There is evidence though to suggest it can have hormonal affects on young boys before they have reached puberty, disrupting their normal hormones. Also, as it affects the central nervous system, which can be beneficial when considered with stress, but it can also be detrimental if used in conjunction with any other type of anaesthesia. Therefore, it is better to not use lavender essential oil if you will be using another type of anaesthetic, such as in the performance of surgery. Also avoid if you have high blood pressure.

Blends well with:

> Bergamot essential oil, cedar wood essential oil, chamomile essential oil, clary sage essential oil, clove essential oil, eucalyptus essential oil, geranium essential oil, grapefruit essential oil, juniper essential oil, lemon essential oil, lemongrass essential oil, mandarin essential oil, marjoram essential oil, oakmoss essential oil, palmarosa essential oil, patchouli essential oil, peppermint essential oil, pine essential oil, ravensara essential oil, rose essential oil, rosemary

essential oil, tea tree essential oil and thyme essential oil.

MARJORAM ESSENTIAL OIL

Marjoram essential oil comes from both the fresh leaves and also dried leaves of a marjoram plant, a herb found in Cyprus and southern Turkey

It is often likened to oregano and is actually quite popular to cook with.

The chemical components of marjoram essential oil include sabinene, alpha-terpinene, gamma-terpinene, cymene, terpinolene, linalool, sabinene hydrate, linalyl acetate, terpineol and gamma terpineol.

The health benefits of marjoram essential oil for arthritis include that it is an analgesic, which reduces pain, inflammation and over-exerted muscles. Its use as a nervine and sedative also complements this as it helps to reduce stress.

There are no real risks known although generally pregnant women are cautioned against its use.

Blends well with:

Bergamot essential oil, cedar wood essential oil, chamomile essential oil, cypress essential oil, eucalyptus essential oil and tea tree essential oil.

MYRRH ESSENTIAL OIL

Myrrh essential oil is extracted from the commiphora myrrh tree and is found in Egypt.

Myrrh has been historically known to be good for arthritis – many have commented on the use of a salve blend using myrrh for alleviation of the discomforting symptoms of arthritis. It was abundantly used in the Middle East and was a known gift to King Solomon from the Queen of Sheba.

The chemical components of myrrh essential oil include alpha-pinene, cadinene, limonene, cuminaldehyde, eugenol, cresol, heerabolene, acetic acid, formic acid and sesquiterpenes.

Myrrh has many medicinal purposes and the essential oil has benefits for arthritis as well. Its anti-inflammatory properties protect arthritis sufferers from severe swelling. It's circulatory and tonic elements mean that the immune system is boosted, problems of which are often associated with arthritis.

Excessive use of myrrh essential oil can be toxic and pregnant women should avoid it as it stimulates the uterus.

Blends well with:

> Frankincense essential oil, lavender essential oil, palma rosa essential oil, patchouli essential oil, rosewood essential oil, sandalwood essential oil, tea tree essential oil and thyme essential oil.

PEPPERMINT ESSENTIAL OIL

Peppermint essential oil is made from the leaves of the peppermint herb native to Europe.

Peppermint or mint has a special story in Greek mythology, which tells of a river nymph called Minthe, being seduced by Hades, but before he could, Persephone, his wife, turned Minthe into a mint plant. Hades apparently softened the spell with the scent now so known, so when people walked past the mint plant, they would smell her sweetness.

The chemical components of peppermint essential oil include menthol, menthone, menthyl acetate, menthofuran and 1,8-cineol.

The menthol in peppermint is a cooling agent, easing the discomfort and pain felt by arthritis sufferers. It also helps to boost the immune system associated with rheumatic arthritis and can alleviate stress by clearing the mind.

Caution should be applied in terms of possible irritation to the skin and patch tests should always be undertaken before application to the skin.

Blends well with:

> Eucalyptus essential oil, rosemary essential oil, lemon essential oil and marjoram essential oil.

ROSEMARY ESSENTIAL OIL

Rosemary essential oil is made from leaves on the rosemary herb found in countries around the Mediterranean.

During years of 1100-1350, rosemary was often made into a wreath and emerged in fragrant water for brides.

The chemical components found in rosemary essential oil include alpha-pinene, borneol, beta-pinene, camphor, bornyl acetate, camphene, 1,8-cineole and limonene.

Rosemary essential oil contains antioxidants that are helpful in tackling arthritis as it helps to remove the body of toxins, applicable to gout and to boost immunity.

The use of rosemary essential oil is advised against if in pregnancy or if you suffer from epilepsy or high blood pressure.

Blends well with:

> Cedar wood essential oil, geranium essential oil, lavender essential oil and peppermint essential oil.

TEA TREE ESSENTIAL OIL

Tea tree essential oil is made from the seed of the tea plant found in Australia.

The tea tree oil itself became popular in the 1920s when an Arthur Penfold, through his research, found that it was incredibly effective as an anti-microbial.

The chemical components of tea tree essential oil include alpha-pinene, beta-pinene, sabinene, myrcene, alpha-phellandrene, alpha-terpinene, limonene, cineole, gamma-terpinene, para-cymene, terpinolene, linalool, terpinenol and alpha-terpineol.

Tea tree essential oil is known for a number of medical properties. However, for arthritis sufferers, tea tree essential oil is beneficial as it stops the swelling in the joints.

Tea tree essential oil is highly toxic and should never be ingested. Its use is only to be applied topically and in a diluted form. Some users may find it is a slight irritant to the skin. It also has drying effects. Therefore, if using this essential oil for psoriasis, try blending tea tree with another essential oil.

Blends well with:

> Cinnamon essential oil, clary sage essential oil, clove essential oil, geranium essential oil, lavender essential oil, lemon essential oil, myrrh essential oil, nutmeg essential oil, rosemary essential oil and thyme essential oil.

THYME ESSENTIAL OIL

Thyme essential oil is made through extraction from the herb, thymus aesvitus, commonly known as 'thyme'.

Thyme is very commonly used in cooking and has often been thought of as an antidote to venom and poison. It was often turned to during the Plague in the 1340s.

The chemical components of thyme essential oil include alpha-thujone, alpha-pinene, camphene, beta-pinene, para-cymene, alpha-terpinene, linalool, borneol, beta-caryophyllene, thymol and carvacrol

It is thymol that has great antiseptic qualities and has been used to treat swelling and inflammations and therefore is a great ingredient used in the treatment of arthritis. However, as a tonic, it also works to boost the immune system.

As with many natural or chemical raw materials, there may be side effects. Thyme can be toxic and is better to be avoided in large quantities. Those in pregnancy should also avoid it. Thyme can be a skin irritant so it always recommended testing the effects of thyme on a small patch of skin first.

Blends well with:

> Bergamot essential oil, grapefruit essential oil, lemon essential oil, lavender essential oil, pine essential oil and rosemary essential oil.

SANDALWOOD ESSENTIAL OIL

Sandalwood essential oil is made from the chips and billets cut from heartwood of the sandalwood tree. There are three types of sandalwood: Indian, Australian and Hawaiian but it is the Indian variety that has health benefits.

Sandalwood is one of the few woods that maintains its pleasing scent and has been prolifically used in cosmetic and fragrance markets and industries.

The main chemical components of sandalwood essential oil are beta-santalol, santyl-acetate and santalene.

The health benefits of the sandalwood essential oil for arthritis are based in its anti-inflammatory properties, sedative and ability to treat lymph nodes and muscle spasms.

There are no known risks to using sandalwood but it is recommended for it not to be used on raw skin. And should always be combined with carrier oil before being applied.

Blends well with:

> Bergamot essential oil, black pepper essential oil, geranium essential oil, lavender essential oil, myrrh essential oil, rose essential oil and ylang-ylang essential oil.

VETIVER ESSENTIAL OIL

Vetiver essential oil comes from vetiver, a type of grass, more commonly known as khus. It is found in India.

Vetiver or khus can be used in construction too. It has a long stem and can typically be used for roof thatching or even mud brick making.

The main chemical components of vetiver essential oil include alpha-vetivone, benzoic acid, beta-vetivone, furfurol, vetivene, vetiverol and vetivenyl vetivenate.

The health benefits of vetiver essential oil for arthritis include it as anti-inflammatory that is used for all types of swelling, particularly of the joints. Its use as a tonic helps to boost the immune system also to help prevent tissue around the joints being attacked in those that suffer from rheumatoid arthritis.

There are no known hazards to vetiver essential oil as it not toxic and does not irritate the skin.

Blends well with:

Benzoin essential oil, grapefruit essential oil, jasmine essential oil, lavender essential oil and ylang-ylang essential oil.

WINTERGREEN ESSENTIAL OIL

Wintergreen essential oil comes from the leaves of the wintergreen tree found in North America.

Native Americans that have used it to alleviate back pain, rheumatism, fever and headaches, have documented the use of oil derived from wintergreen.

The chemical components of wintergreen essential oil include gaultherilene and menthyl salicylate.

The health benefits of wintergreen essential oil for arthritis includes it being an analgesic, which means it is used for pain relief. This is a well know benefit of wintergreen and you only need to rub it into the skin for it to absorb and start working. It is also anti-rheumatic and anti-arthritic. External application means it is absorbed into the tissues and muscles surrounding affected joints to aid the circulation of blood in that area. It also prevents uric acid from entering the area and acts as a diuretic to prevent the build of uric acid further in the joints.

Application of wintergreen should be done with caution as over application would result in the build up of menthyl salicylate entering the blood stream, which can be fatal. If ingested it is poisonous and can cause damage to internal organs.

Blends well with:

Mint essential oil, narcissus essential oil, oregano essential oil, thyme essential oil, vanilla essential oil and ylang-ylang essential oil.

YARROW ESSENTIAL OIL

Yarrow essential oil comes from a herb in its dried form found in Europe.

Ancient Greek legend has it that Achilles, the hero of the Trojan War, used the yarrow herb to help heal the tendon in his Achilles – Achilles heel.

The chemical components of yarrow essential oil include alpha-pinene, borneol acetate, borneol, beta-pinene, camphene, camphor, cineole, chamazulene, gamma-terpinene, limonene, isoartemisia ketone, sabinene and tricyclene.

The health benefits of yarrow essential oil for arthritis are well known as an anti-inflammatory and is also known for being anti-rheumatic so it increases circulation, preventing the build-up of uric acid, common in arthritic patients. Its use as a tonic is used to boost the immune system and it has calming properties in addition.

Cautionary notes include proneness to headaches and irritation to the skin after long-term use or high dosages. Avoid ingesting during pregnancy.

Blends well with:

Angelica essential oil, cedar wood essential oil, oak moss essential oil and verbena essential oil.

CHAPTER 4

COMPLEMENTARY SUPPLEMENTS

Using essential oil for treatment of arthritis clearly has historical precedence and the benefits are commonly known, particularly with regards to absorption into the joints to reduce swelling. However, there are many supplements that can complement the application of essential oils and knowing a little more about them individually can be helpful.

CARRIER OILS

Firstly, essential oils should never be applied directly to the skin due to their volatility.

Carrier oils are vegetable based oils that are used to dilute the essential oil before it is applied directly to the skin. Essential oils may cause irritation to some skin types, therefore, it is never recommended to apply it without mixing it with a base.

Carrier oils will be less volatile and relatively neutral in smell. They can also have healing properties themselves; therefore, their use with essential oils for the treatment of arthritis can be very beneficial.

Carrier oils known to help arthritis, when combined with essential oils, include:

Emu, hemp, jojoba, pomegranate, sweet almond and tamanu. This is due to their anti-inflammatory properties.

Emu Oil

Emu oil is an atypical carrier oil as it is not vegetable based. Emu oil is taken from the fat of the Emu bird. It works for arthritis as it contains fatty acids that help reduce pain and swelling.

Hemp Oil

Hemp oil is extracted from the hemp plant and its fatty acids and polyunsaturated fats help the healing process and work to reduce pain and inflammation.

Jojoba Oil

Jojoba oil is derived from the jojoba shrub native to California. It is a great oil to use for arthritis as the myristic acid within it has anti-inflammatory effects.

Pomegranate Seed Oil

Pomegranate seed oil comes from the fruit, pomegranate. Studies have shown that the extract taken from the pomegranate can help reduce inflammation, which makes it an excellent aid to complement a number of essential oils.

Sweet Almond Oil

Sweet almond oil comes from the seeds of the sweet almond tree. Sweet almond oil is a good carrier for essential oil treatments for arthritis for its ability to reduce inflammation.

Tamanu Oil

Tamanu oil is extracted by pressing the nuts of the calophyllum inophyllum or the calophyllum tacamahaca tree, found in many parts of Asia. Tamanu oil can help arthritis as it has anti-inflammatory and anti-oxidant properties that reduces swelling and removes toxins in order to boost immunity.

Other Supplements

Aloe Vera

Aloe Vera is a stemless plant found throughout the world. Aloe vera's usefulness in the treatment of arthritis is two-fold. Firstly, it has been known to reduce inflammation, although evidence for this is mostly anecdotal.

Secondly, if you are using prescribed treatment, such as the use of NSAIDs, mentioned in chapter 1, then side effects can cause stomach problems. Aloe vera can help to soothe stomach problems associated with such treatments.

Mustard Seed

The mustard seed is the seed from the mustard plant found in the sub-continent. It has its use in relieving joint pain and can be applied topically as an external treatment, for example in a salve or through an oil, the heat from which helps to improve the circulation of blood.

However, it can also be taken orally, as the magnesium, selenium and fatty acids that it contains can improve many symptoms associated with arthritis.

Olive Oil

While olive oil, derived from the fruit of the olive, can be used as a carrier oil alongside essential oils, it can also be taken orally.

Olive oil contains the compound oleocanthal, which acts as an anti-inflammatory as it reduces the COX1 and COX2 enzymes that cause inflammation. In particular substitute other fats used in cooking such as butter.

Cayenne

Cayenne pepper, which can come in a powdered form, comes from the capsicum family. Cayenne's benefit to arthritis is three-fold. Firstly, it helps blood flow, removing toxins and preventing the build up of uric acid.

Better circulation is also good for the immune system.

Secondly, it is a pain relief and can help arthritic patients feel more comfortable. It could be used as part of an ointment or external application as well as being used in cooking.

Thirdly, it has a counter-irritant affect, causing irritation to the tissue but distracting from the more severe joint pain.

CHAPTER 5

RECIPES

Recipe 1 – Cayenne, ginger and mustard seed massage oil

1 tbsp. cayenne pepper

2 tbsp. crushed mustard seeds

10 drops ginger essential oil

250 ml sunflower oil

Combine ingredients and leave them in a jar for one week to allow all of the properties to infuse. After a week, you can strain the oil and you are left with a great massage oil to use on joint pain.

Recipe 2 – Arthritic back pain remedy

5 drops chamomile essential oil and 5 drops lavender essential oil

Or

5 drops clary sage essential oil and 5 drops frankincense essential oil

Or

5 drops rosemary essential oil and 5 drops peppermint essential oil

Or

5 drops ginger essential oil and 5 drops yarrow essential oil

1 oz jojoba oil

The union of these essential oils combines the anti-inflammatory properties with greater circulation and mobility i.e. reducing stiffness.

Combine the chosen blend with the jojoba and massage on your lower back. You can use it up to two times daily.

Alternatively just drop the essential oil blends into a bath, for aromatic arthritic bathe.

Recipe 3 – Juniper Ointment

10 drops juniper essential oil

2 cups carrier oil (olive oil, sweet almond oil or jojoba oil is best)

2 – 3 tbsp. beeswax

Add the beeswax to a bowl over boiling water and add the juniper essential oil and carrier oil of choice. Once melted, pour into jars and allow to set. Apply to affected areas.

Recipe 4 – Bath soak

10 drops essential oil of choice

1 oz carrier oil of choice

2-3 cups Epsom salts

Combine the essential oil with the carrier oil and then add to the bath. Add the Epsom salts, last.

Recipe 5 – Hot Compress

4 drops essential oil of choice

1 pint hot water

Small towel

Add the essential oil to the hot water and place the towel on top of the hot water, allowing it to soak up (not so hot that you can't take it). Squeeze any excess off and place the compress over affected painful joints.

Recipe 6 – Pain Relieving Peppermint and Eucalyptus Oil Blend

5-10 drops peppermint essential oil

5-10 drops eucalyptus essential oil

1-2 tbsp. carrier oil (choose olive oil or sweet almond)

Dark bottle

This blend is specifically for pain relief.

Blend the essential oils together, adding the carrier oil. Store it in a bottle or apply immediately to the affected areas. Keep away from the light.

Recipe 7 – Soothing Rub

Glass container

2 oz fractionated coconut oil

6 drops tea tree essential oil

6 drops rosemary essential oil

6 drops lavender essential oil

This blend combines anti-inflammatory properties with pain relief and a scent for a soothing mood. Combine all of the ingredients together for a complete rub. Store in a jar away from the light.

Recipe 8 – Pain Cream

1 cup coconut oil

10 drops valor

10 drop panaway

10 drops peppermint essential oil

Combine all of these ingredients together for a pain relief cream to use on arthritic joints.

Recipe 9 - Knee Relief

12 drops clove essential oil

2 oz carrier oil of choice

Combine these ingredients to create a 1% dilution mix. Massage the blend into your knee for relief from arthritic pain of the knee. This should be the right dilution to avoid any skin irritation.

Recipe 10 – Spinal Column Blend

15-20 drops peppermint essential oil

15-20 drops ginger essential oil

15-20 drops black pepper essential oil

15-20 drops juniper essential oil

15-20 drops eucalyptus essential oil

Carrier oil of choice

4 oz bottle

Add all of the oils to the bottle and fill the bottle up with the carrier oil. You can apply this to your spinal column but it is not meant for a general massage oil for any part of your body, it is specifically for your spinal column as it is a high concentration blend of 5%.

CHAPTER 6

MAKING SENSE OF IT ALL

Utilising essential oils for arthritis is well documented. Many of the properties contained in the essential oils address symptoms commonly associated with arthritis. That is they reduce inflammation, they relieve pain, increase blood circulation, remove toxins and boost immunity. They can also help alleviate stress so one's mind as well as body can be taken care of.

A large number of individuals have opted for essential oils to take care of their arthritic condition. There are many organisations, forums and blogs that are dedicated to this area of treatment for different arthritic conditions, which should be evidence to its usefulness. The dilemma can only be to choose which one.

There are 22 listed essential oils in this book that have properties that are extremely beneficial to the treatment of arthritis. However, the most cited oils are frankincense, myrrh, cedar wood, yarrow and wintergreen. These essential oils are extremely effective at reducing inflammation. There are some slightly more common essential oils however, such as rosemary, lavender and peppermint. They are more accessible and most probably more affordable.

However, it is personal choice to some degree, and is dependent on your symptoms. You should consider the main symptoms you are exhibiting and which oils have been highlighted for those specific symptoms. Gout should be looked at with a view to choosing those essential oils that have properties for removing toxins so as to stop uric acid building up in the joints. It's quite useful to combine essential oils so that you complement those that are known for reducing swelling and those that relive pain or boost immunity, so on and so forth. Osteoarthritis may warrant the use of grapefruit essential oil to help stop stiffness. Some of the secondary symptoms may need to be addressed also – lack of energy, weak muscles or weight gain, which may lead to high blood pressure or diabetes etc. The list of healing properties and chemical components of each essential oil recommended for arthritis should provide you with the data you need to make informed choices.

Consider also the side effects – you may start to notice a trend in what suits you and the best method to apply them as well as what doesn't!

It is advised to try a few and notice the short-term and long-term results.

Chapter 5 provides some recipe examples; however, you can experiment as long as the precautions are followed. Different combinations of essential oils as well as carrier oils can be tried and tested until one suits you and has the desired affect on your arthritis.

Please be cautious of the strength and concentration of the essential oils you use. It is recommended that you generally stick to a 1% concentration, which is 10 drops of essential oil for every one ounce of carrier oil. The more severe the symptoms, the greater the concentration you may wish to apply; however, advice should always be sought.

Essential oils are not without its side effects so proceed with caution. The application of essential oils does not need a lot of equipment; however, if you become an avid user of essential oils to treat psoriasis or other aspects of your health, then you may want to invest in some small jars, droppers or a diffuser. The mixing of ingredients can be done using normal kitchen equipment. When making up recipes or storing essential oils, keep away from heat and light, as this will cause the oils to break down. Use dark bottles and refrigerate where possible.

There are dedicated homeopathy stores that may sell all of the equipment as well as the essential oils you want to use. All businesses are nowadays listed on the internet, therefore, a quick search will reveal your local store and it may be worth having a browse. Some essential oils can be expensive so it is worth looking at comparable prices on the internet – they can all be ordered online. The added benefit of hopping down to the store is that you will save on delivery costs and you have the bonus of being able to speak to a homoeopathist one on one.

CONCLUSION

Thank you again for purchasing and reading this book!

I hope this book was able to help you to understand more about the essential oils available for arthritis and how and when to use them.

The next step is to start trying out those suggested essential oils to help lead you to relief and recovery.

Finally, if you enjoyed this book, then I'd like to ask you for a favor, would you be kind enough to leave a review for this book on Amazon? It'd be greatly appreciated!

Thank you and good luck!

57232496R00042

Made in the USA
Middletown, DE
16 December 2017